# GLORIOUSTINA ESSIA

# The World of Herbal Medicine

*Tracing the Journey from Ancient Roots to Modern Integration*

First edition

This book was professionally typeset on Reedsy.
Find out more at reedsy.com

# Contents

# Introduction to Book 1: The World of Herbal Medicine

In this foundational section of "Green Healing: The Natural Medicine Bible," we explore herbal medicine's rich and varied world. "The World of Herbal Medicine" is more than just a glimpse into a field of healing; it's a voyage across time and cultures, a dive into the science behind nature's remedies, and an examination of the intricate relationship between plants and human health.

From ancient civilizations to modern integrative health clinics, herbal medicine has been a cornerstone of healing practices worldwide. Each chapter in this section delves deep into the roots of herbalism, tracing its evolution through history, understanding its resurgence in the contemporary world, and unraveling the scientific basis that underpins its efficacy.

We begin by looking back at the dawn of herbal healing, understanding how our ancestors used plants daily for healing and wellness. This historical perspective provides a backdrop for the practice of herbal medicine and highlights its enduring relevance.

As we move forward, we will explore how herbal medicine is perceived and practiced today in a world where technology and traditional knowledge intersect. The chapters will illuminate the challenges and triumphs in integrating herbal medicine with modern healthcare systems and how this integration impacts patient care and wellness strategies.

The science behind herbal remedies is a fascinating and crucial aspect of this journey. We will uncover the active compounds in herbs, delve into significant scientific research, and address the challenges faced in validating herbal medicine in the scientific community.

Finally, we will take a global tour of herbal traditions, celebrating the cultural diversity in herbal practices. This panoramic view enriches our understanding and fosters a deep appreciation for how different cultures have embraced and evolved with herbal medicine.

"The World of Herbal Medicine" is your gateway into the vast and vibrant realm of herbal healing. Whether you are a curious beginner, a seasoned practitioner, or simply someone interested in the natural ways of wellness, these chapters offer a comprehensive and enlightening journey through one of humanity's oldest and most trusted forms of healing.

# CHAPTER 1: HISTORY AND EVOLUTION OF HERBAL MEDICINE

## The Dawn of Herbal Healing

The dawn of herbal healing marks the genesis of humankind's journey with medicinal plants, a voyage deeply intertwined with our earliest cultural and survival instincts. Rooted in the ancient soils of human history, this primal connection reflects an intuitive understanding that nature held potent remedies within its flora.

In these nascent stages, every tribe and early civilization, from the lush valleys of the Nile to the dense forests of the Amazon, discovered the healing powers of their local herbs. These discoveries were not mere chance but a result of keen observation, trial and error, and a deep understanding of the natural world.

Shamans, healers, and medicine men and women were the custodians of this sacred knowledge. They observed the effects of herbs on animals, experimented with their uses, and passed down their knowledge orally through generations. This Era was characterized by a holistic approach, where healing was physical and spiritual, with herbs playing a role in rituals and ceremonies.

This Era set the foundation for all traditional medicine systems, whether it's Ayurveda in India, which classifies herbs based on their effects on body energies, or Traditional Chinese Medicine, which incorporates herbs into a complex system of balance and harmony. These ancient practices, rich in wisdom and experience, laid the groundwork for the diverse and sophisticated herbal healing practices we see worldwide today.

This period is a testament to the enduring bond between humans and the plant kingdom, a relationship of mutual respect and survival, where plants nourished and healed, forming an integral part of the human journey through the ages.

## Traditional Chinese Medicine (TCM)

Traditional Chinese Medicine (TCM) is a holistic health and wellness system practised in China for thousands of years. Rooted in ancient Taoist philosophy, TCM views the human body as a miniature version of the universe governed by the same laws and elements. It is based on the concept of Qi (vital energy), which flows through the body along meridian pathways.

TCM encompasses various modalities, including herbal medicine, acupuncture, massage (tui na), exercise (qigong), and dietary therapy. The practice is fundamentally about maintaining or restoring balance and harmony within and between the body and its environment.

Herbal medicine is a cornerstone of TCM, involving a complex system of plant-based treatments. Herbs in TCM are selected and combined based on their properties, such as taste, temperature, and the organs or meridians they target. These formulations are tailored to the individual's unique imbalance of Yin (passive, cooling energy) and Yang (active, warming energy) to treat symptoms and the cause of illness.

TCM practitioners also focus on the prevention of disease and the promotion of health, not just the treatment of illness. Diagnosis in TCM involves:

- Observing the patient's tongue.
- Checking the pulse.
- Considering other physical and emotional signs and symptoms in the context of their environment and lifestyle.

TCM's approach to health and disease is distinct from Western medicine, emphasizing a holistic view of the body and its place in the natural world. This ancient practice continues to evolve and is recognized and used globally, often in conjunction with modern medical treatments.

## Ayurveda

Ayurveda, an ancient Indian system of medicine, dates back over 3,000 years and is one of the world's oldest holistic healing systems. Its name comes from the Sanskrit words "Ayur" (life) and "Veda" (science or knowledge), literally translating to the "science of life."

At the heart of Ayurveda is the concept of balance within the body, mind, and spirit, achieved through a combination of diet, lifestyle practices, and herbal remedies. It emphasizes the prevention of disease, rejuvenation of the body, and the extension of life span.

The practice of Ayurveda is founded on the theory of five elements (earth, water, fire, air, ether) that manifest in the human body as three fundamental energies or doshas: Vata (air and space – controls movement), Pitta (fire and water – controls metabolism), and Kapha (water and earth – controls structure and fluid balance). Every individual has a unique combination of these doshas, which defines their constitution and health tendencies.

Ayurvedic treatment is highly individualized and begins with assessing a person's unique dosha balance. Herbal remedies are a key component of Ayurveda and are chosen based on their ability to balance the particular doshas that are out of alignment in the individual. These remedies often include a variety of herbs, minerals, and metals and are administered in conjunction with lifestyle adjustments and dietary changes.

Ayurveda includes detoxification and purification procedures (Panchakarma), yoga, meditation, and massage therapy (Abhyanga) as integral parts of the healing process. These practices aim not only at treating diseases but also at maintaining and improving health and wellness.

Ayurveda offers a rich, holistic framework for understanding and treating the human body, emphasizing harmony between the individual and the natural world and a deep connection between physical health and emotional, spiritual, and mental well-being.

## Indigenous Practices

Indigenous practices in herbal medicine refer to the rich and diverse healing traditions developed by indigenous communities worldwide. These practices are deeply rooted in a holistic understanding of health, where life's physical, spiritual, emotional, and environmental aspects are intimately connected.

A profound knowledge of local flora characterizes Indigenous herbalism, passed down through generations orally or through hands-on apprenticeships. Healers, often known as shamans, medicine men or women, or herbalists, play a crucial role in these communities, acting as the custodians of medicinal plant knowledge and healing rituals.

**Key aspects of indigenous herbal practices include:**

- **Deep Connection with Nature:** Indigenous herbalism is based on a profound spiritual relationship with the land and its plants. It involves understanding the intricate balance of ecosystems and the belief that plants possess spirits or energies that can aid healing.
- **Holistic Healing Approaches:** These practices often encompass more than just physical healing, addressing emotional and spiritual well-being. Rituals, ceremonies, and storytelling are frequently integral parts of the healing process.
- **Local and Seasonal Herbs:** Indigenous healers use plants readily available in their immediate environment, focusing on seasonal and locally abundant herbs. This local focus ensures a deep understanding of each plant's characteristics and uses.
- **Sustainable Practices:** There is a strong emphasis on sustainable harvesting methods that respect and preserve the natural abundance of medicinal plants, ensuring they continue to thrive for future generations.

Indigenous herbal practices vary greatly from region to region, reflecting the diversity of the world's ecosystems and cultures. From the use of ayahuasca in Amazonian tribes to the wide array of medicinal plants used by Native Americans, each tradition offers a unique perspective on health and healing.

These practices have contributed significantly to modern pharmacology, with many commonly used drugs derived from plants first used in indigenous medicine. Today, there is a growing recognition of the value of these traditional healing practices, not only for their direct health benefits but also for their approach to wellness and harmony with nature.

## Herbalism Through the Ages

Herbalism's journey through history is as rich and diverse as the plants it studies. From ancient to today, using plants for medicinal purposes has been a common thread in human civilization.

## Ancient Civilizations

The earliest records of herbal medicine come from ancient civilizations like the Egyptians, Chinese, Indians, and Greeks. These cultures had extensive knowledge of medicinal plants, documented in texts like the Ebers Papyrus (Egypt) and Charaka Samhita (India).

## Middle Ages

During the Middle Ages in Europe, monasteries preserved and advanced the knowledge of herbal medicine. Monks cultivated medicinal gardens and produced texts, blending Greco-Roman knowledge with local herbal traditions.

## Renaissance

The Renaissance revived interest in scientific inquiry and natural history, leading to more detailed study and documentation of plants. This era saw the birth of modern botany and increased global exchange of medicinal plant knowledge.

## Colonialism and Global Exchange

As Europeans explored and colonized other parts of the world, they encountered new medicinal plants and integrated them into their pharmacopoeia. This period was marked by a significant exchange of herbal knowledge between different cultures.

## 19th and 20th Centuries

The Industrial Revolution and advances in chemistry led to the isolation of active compounds from plants and the rise of synthetic pharmaceuticals. However, herbal medicine continued to be practised in rural and indigenous communities.

## Contemporary Revival

In recent decades, there has been a resurgence of interest in herbal medicine as part of the holistic health movement. Today, herbalism is a vibrant field, blending traditional knowledge with modern scientific research and practised as a complement to and an alternative to conventional medicine.

Throughout the ages, herbalism has adapted to the changing landscapes of science, culture, and medicine, proving its enduring relevance and importance in the quest for health and well-being.

# The Intersection with Modern Medicine

The intersection of herbal and modern medicine is a complex and evolving relationship marked by collaboration and tension. As medical science has advanced, the role and perception of herbal remedies have undergone significant changes.

## Early Confrontations

In the early stages of modern medicine, especially with the rise of synthetic pharmaceuticals in the 19th and 20th centuries, herbal medicine often conflicted with the emerging scientific approach to health. The preference for standardized, laboratory-produced medications overshadowed the traditional use of plant-based remedies.

## Integration and Complementary Use

More recently, there has been a growing interest in integrating herbal medicine with conventional medical practices. This is seen in the rise of complementary and alternative medicine (CAM), where herbal treatments are used alongside or adjunct to standard medical treatments, often for chronic conditions, wellness, and preventive care.

## Scientific Validation

The modern era has also brought a scientific lens to the study of medicinal plants. Numerous studies and clinical trials are conducted to understand the efficacy, safety, and mechanisms of action of herbal remedies. This research has led to the validation of many traditional uses of herbs, although challenges in standardization and quality control remain.

## Holistic and Patient-Centered Approaches

The rise of patient-centred care and holistic health perspectives in modern medicine has further fueled interest in herbal medicine. Patients and health-care practitioners are increasingly looking at health and wellness in a more integrated manner, considering physical, mental, and emotional well-being, where herbal medicine often plays a key role.

## Global and Traditional Knowledge Systems

Modern medicine increasingly recognizes the value of traditional knowledge systems, including indigenous and folk medicine practices. There's a growing understanding that these systems offer valuable insights and approaches to health that can complement modern medical practices.

The intersection of herbal and modern medicine represents an ongoing dialogue between tradition and innovation. This relationship continues to evolve, shaped by scientific advancements, cultural shifts, and a growing emphasis on holistic and integrative approaches to health and wellness.

# The Future of Herbal Medicine

The future of herbal medicine looks promising, blending traditional knowledge with modern scientific advancements and a growing global consciousness about health and wellness.

- **Scientific Advancements and Research:** Continued research in phyto-chemistry and pharmacognosy is expected to unlock deeper insights into how plant compounds interact with the human body. This will likely lead to more effective and targeted use of herbal remedies, including personalized medicine approaches based on genetic profiles.
- **Integration in Mainstream Healthcare:** Herbal medicine is poised to

become more integrated into mainstream healthcare systems. This integration might include a greater emphasis on herbal education in medical training, more collaboration between herbalists and conventional healthcare providers, and an increase in clinical trials assessing the efficacy of herbal treatments.

- **Technological Innovations:** Advances in technology, such as AI and data analytics, could revolutionize how herbal medicines are researched, developed, and prescribed. These technologies might enable more precise dosage recommendations and a better understanding of herb-drug interactions.

- **Sustainable Practices and Biodiversity Conservation:** As the demand for herbal remedies grows, sustainable cultivation and ethical sourcing of medicinal plants will become increasingly important. This focus on sustainability will help preserve plant biodiversity and ensure that herbal medicine remains a viable practice for future generations.

- **Globalization and Cross-Cultural Exchange:** The globalization of herbal medicine will likely continue, facilitating a rich exchange of knowledge and practices between different cultures. This exchange could lead to discovering new medicinal plants and a broader acceptance of diverse healing traditions.

- **Regulatory Developments:** Enhanced regulation and standardization of herbal products are expected, improving their safety, quality, and efficacy. This could increase public trust and more widespread use of herbal remedies.

The future of herbal medicine is one of potential and growth, characterized by a harmonious blend of tradition and innovation and a deeper integration into the fabric of global healthcare and wellness practices.

# CHAPTER 2: UNDERSTANDING HERBAL MEDICINE TODAY

## Defining Herbal Medicine

Herbal medicine today is characterized by using plants and their extracts for therapeutic purposes. It encompasses a broad spectrum:

- **Traditional Practices:** Rooted in ancient wisdom, these practices involve using herbs based on centuries-old knowledge passed down through generations. Each culture has unique herbal traditions, often closely tied to local flora and historical uses.
- **Modern Evidence-Based Approaches:** This aspect of herbal medicine relies on contemporary scientific research to understand and validate the efficacy and safety of herbal treatments. It includes clinical trials and pharmacological studies of plant compounds.

## Global Perspectives

The practice of herbal medicine varies greatly around the world, reflecting cultural, historical, and ecological diversity:

- **Primary Healthcare in Many Cultures:** In several regions, particularly Asia, Africa, and South America, herbal medicine remains a primary form of healthcare, deeply ingrained in local customs.

- **Complementary and Alternative Medicine (CAM):** In Western countries, herbal medicine often complements conventional treatments. People increasingly turn to herbal remedies for wellness, preventive care, and chronic conditions that don't respond well to conventional treatments.
- **Cross-Cultural Exchange:** The globalization of herbal medicine has led to an exchange of knowledge and practices, enriching the field with diverse healing traditions and a broader range of medicinal plants.

## The Role of Herbalism in Contemporary Healthcare

Herbal medicine's role in contemporary healthcare is multifaceted, balancing between traditional practices and modern clinical settings:

- **Integrative Healthcare Approach:** Herbal remedies are increasingly being integrated into mainstream healthcare. This includes hospitals and clinics offering CAM therapies alongside conventional treatments, recognizing the benefits of a holistic approach.
- **Collaboration with Medical Practitioners:** There's growing collaboration between herbalists and conventional healthcare providers. This synergy aims to provide patients with comprehensive care that combines the best of both worlds.
- **Public and Professional Perception:** The perception of herbal medicine has shifted significantly. More healthcare professionals are acknowledging the potential benefits of herbal treatments, especially for chronic conditions, preventive health, and overall wellness.

## Consumer Trends and Self-Care

Several factors drive the rise in consumer interest in herbal medicine:

- **Natural Health Movement:** A growing number of people are turning to natural and organic products, including herbal remedies, as a lifestyle choice towards healthier, more sustainable living.

- **Self-Care and Wellness:** There's an increasing focus on self-care and wellness, with individuals seeking proactive ways to maintain health and well-being. Herbal products like supplements, teas, and essential oils are popular for their perceived safety and natural origins.
- **Information Accessibility:** The internet has made it easier for consumers to access information about herbal remedies, although this also raises concerns about the accuracy and reliability of some sources.

## Scientific Research and Evidence-Based Practice

Scientific research plays a crucial role in modern herbal medicine:

- **Clinical Trials and Studies:** There's a growing body of scientific literature on the efficacy and safety of herbal remedies. Clinical trials and pharmacological research help validate traditional uses and understand the mechanisms behind the healing properties of herbs.
- **Challenges in Research:** Standardizing herbal treatments for research purposes can be challenging due to the complex nature of plant compounds. Additionally, funding and interest in herbal research are often less compared to pharmaceutical drugs.

## Regulatory Environment and Quality Control

The regulatory landscape for herbal medicine is evolving:

- **Quality Control and Standardization:** As the herbal medicine market grows, so does the need for stringent quality control and standardization to ensure product safety and efficacy. This includes accurate labelling, verifying the purity of ingredients, and ensuring that products are free from contaminants.
- **Regulatory Bodies and Policies:** Different countries have varying regulations governing the sale and use of herbal products. In some places, herbs

are regulated like food supplements; in others, they are treated more like medicines, requiring rigorous testing and approval processes.

- **Emerging Technologies and Research Methodologies:** Advanced technologies like genomics, bioinformatics, and AI are beginning to play a role in herbal medicine research. These technologies can help identify active compounds, understand their mechanisms of action, and predict their effects on the human body. This could lead to more personalized and effective herbal treatments.

- **Educational Initiatives:** With the growing interest in herbal medicine, there's a corresponding increase in educational programs and resources. This includes university courses, online platforms, and public workshops to provide accurate information and training for practitioners and consumers. This education is crucial for the safe and effective use of herbal remedies.

- **Global Health Perspectives:** As the world becomes more interconnected, there's an opportunity to learn from different herbal medicine traditions. This global perspective diversifies the range of available treatments and promotes a more inclusive approach to health and wellness.

- **Future Challenges:** The future of herbal medicine will involve addressing challenges such as ensuring sustainable sourcing of medicinal plants, protecting traditional knowledge rights, and navigating the complex landscape of international regulations.

- **Potential for Healthcare Systems:** Herbal medicine has the potential to contribute significantly to global health systems, offering cost-effective, accessible, and holistic treatment options. Its integration into primary healthcare could especially benefit regions with limited access to conventional medicine.

Understanding herbal medicine today requires a multifaceted approach that respects its historical roots, embraces current scientific research, and anticipates future developments and challenges. As it evolves, herbal medicine promises to play an increasingly significant role in global health and wellness.

# CHAPTER 3: THE SCIENCE BEHIND HERBAL REMEDIES

Herbal remedies, deeply rooted in ancient traditions, are increasingly validated by modern science. This chapter delves into the scientific principles underpinning these remedies, highlighting how research unravels the complexities of herbal medicine.

## Understanding Active Compounds in Herbs

Herbal remedies derive their therapeutic properties from various bioactive compounds present in plants. These compounds range from vitamins and minerals to more complex molecules like alkaloids, flavonoids, and terpenes.

- **Alkaloids:** Found in plants like the opium poppy (Papaver somniferum) and goldenseal (Hydrastis canadensis), alkaloids have a wide range of pharmacological effects. Morphine, an alkaloid from the opium poppy, is well-known for its analgesic properties.
- **Flavonoids:** These compounds, found in fruits, vegetables, and herbs like Ginkgo biloba and St. John's Wort (Hypericum perforatum), are known for their antioxidant properties. They help in combating oxidative stress, a factor in many chronic diseases.
- **Terpenes:** These aromatic compounds, found in herbs like peppermint (Mentha piperita) and cannabis (Cannabis sativa), have various therapeutic properties, including anti-inflammatory and analgesic effects.

# Scientific Research and Evidence

The efficacy of herbal remedies is increasingly supported by scientific research, including in vitro (test tube) studies, animal studies, and human clinical trials.

- **Clinical Trials:** Trials on St. John's Wort, for example, have shown its effectiveness in treating mild to moderate depression. Similarly, trials on Ginkgo biloba indicate its potential to improve cognitive function.
- **Mechanisms of Action:** Research aims to understand how these herbs work at a molecular level. For instance, the anti-inflammatory properties of turmeric (Curcuma longa) are attributed to its active compound, curcumin, which inhibits certain molecular pathways involved in inflammation.

# Challenges and Progress in Herbal Research

Researching herbal remedies presents unique challenges compared to conventional pharmaceuticals.

- **Complexity of Plant Compounds:** Unlike single-compound drugs, herbs contain myriad compounds that can interact synergistically, making it difficult to pinpoint the exact mechanism of action. For example, the therapeutic effect of Echinacea in enhancing immune function is due to a combination of its multiple active constituents.
- **Standardization and Quality Control:** The concentration of active plant ingredients can vary based on soil quality, climate, and harvesting methods. This variability poses challenges in standardizing herbal products for research and therapeutic use.
- **Placebo Effect and Double-Blind Studies:** Conducting double-masked studies with herbal remedies can be challenging, especially when the taste and smell of the herb are distinctive. Researchers must find ways to ensure that placebo treatments are convincingly similar to the actual herb being tested.

# Bridging Traditional Knowledge and Modern Science

Modern herbal research often involves bridging traditional knowledge with scientific methodologies.

- **Ethnobotany:** This field studies how different cultures use plants for medicinal purposes, providing valuable insights for scientific research. For instance, using willow bark for pain relief in various cultures led to the discovery of aspirin.
- **Pharmacognosy:** This branch of pharmacology that studies medicinal plants is crucial in identifying new drugs. For example, the cancer drug paclitaxel was originally derived from the Pacific yew tree (Taxus brevifolia), a plant used by indigenous tribes.

# Future Directions in Herbal Medicine Research

The future of herbal medicine research is promising, with several potential directions:

- **Genetic and 'Omics' Technologies:** Advances in genomics, proteomics, and metabolomics offer new ways to understand the complex interactions between herbal compounds and biological systems.
- **Personalized Medicine:** There's potential for using genetic information to tailor herbal treatments to individual patients, optimizing efficacy and minimizing side effects.
- **Integrative Approaches:** Combining herbal remedies with other treatments, like conventional drugs or lifestyle interventions, could lead to more holistic and effective healthcare strategies.

In conclusion, the science behind herbal remedies is a fascinating and rapidly evolving field, bridging ancient wisdom with modern research methodologies. While challenges remain, the potential for herbal medicine to contribute significantly to health and wellness is immense. Continued research and collaboration between traditional practitioners and modern scientists are key to unlocking the full potential of these natural healing agents, paving the way for more effective, safe, and personalized therapeutic options in medicine.

# CHAPTER 4: THE ROLE OF HERBS IN MODERN MEDICINE

As we delve into the intricate world of herbal medicine and its place in the modern medical landscape, it becomes apparent that the role of herbs is not just a relic of traditional practices but a vital, evolving component of contemporary healthcare. This comprehensive exploration seeks to illuminate the multifaceted role of herbs in modern medicine, examining their use in complementary and alternative therapies, the juxtaposition with pharmaceuticals, and real-world examples of their integration.

## Complementary and Alternative Medicine (CAM)

In recent years, there has been a significant surge in the popularity of Complementary and Alternative Medicine (CAM), with herbal medicine taking a prominent place. CAM refers to a wide range of practices and products not traditionally part of conventional medicine. Herbs in CAM are often used in a preventive capacity, aiming to maintain health and wellness rather than solely treat disease.

## Integrative Health Approaches

Integrative health combines conventional medical treatments with CAM practices that have shown some high-quality evidence of safety and effectiveness. This approach is gaining traction, particularly in managing chronic conditions where conventional medicine alone does not offer complete relief or when patients seek more natural treatment methods. For instance, St. John's Wort is commonly used in integrative therapy for mild to moderate depression, and Ginkgo biloba is often recommended for cognitive impairment.

## Herbs vs. Pharmaceuticals

The relationship between herbal remedies and pharmaceutical drugs is complex and multifaceted.

### Efficacy and Safety

One of the key differences lies in the approach to treatment. Pharmaceuticals typically contain single, highly concentrated active ingredients designed for targeted action. In contrast, herbal remedies are compounds that work synergistically, often producing more holistic effects with fewer side effects. However, the efficacy of herbal remedies can vary due to factors like the quality of raw materials and methods of preparation.

### Side Effects

While pharmaceuticals are often associated with a list of potential side effects, herbs are generally perceived as safer. However, this is only sometimes the case; herbs can interact with other medications and be potent. Hence, the need for professional guidance in their use cannot be overstated.

## Case Studies: Integration in Modern Practices

Example 1: Herbal Oncology

In oncology, certain herbs are used alongside chemotherapy to alleviate side effects and improve the patient's quality of life. For instance, ginger is often recommended to manage nausea associated with chemotherapy.

Example 2: Cardiology

In cardiology, hawthorn is a herb used alongside conventional heart medications to treat heart failure, with studies showing benefits in symptom control and physiological outcomes.

Example 3: Mental Health

In mental health, herbal supplements like valerian root for insomnia and anxiety have been used effectively, providing a more gentle alternative to conventional sedatives.

## The Future of Herbs in Modern Medicine

Integrating herbal medicine into mainstream healthcare seems promising as we look to the future. This is driven by increasing patient interest, growing scientific evidence supporting the efficacy of herbal treatments, and a broader shift towards more holistic, patient-centred care models. Moreover, the rise of multidisciplinary research in pharmacognosy (the study of medicines derived from natural sources) is helping to bridge the gap between traditional herbal wisdom and modern scientific understanding.

In conclusion, the role of herbs in modern medicine is dynamic and expanding. We can look forward to a more holistic, effective, and personalized healthcare system with a balanced approach that respects both the power and limitations of herbal remedies and integrates the best practices from conventional and herbal medicine.

# CHAPTER 5: GLOBAL HERBAL TRADITIONS

Global herbal traditions encompass a rich and diverse tapestry of practices and beliefs, each deeply rooted in different societies' cultural and historical contexts.

## Cultural Diversity in Herbal Practices

Herbal medicine traditions vary greatly across cultures, reflecting local flora, historical influences, and indigenous knowledge.

- **Asian Traditions:** In countries like China and India, herbal medicine is integral to Traditional Chinese Medicine (TCM) and Ayurveda. TCM uses a complex system of herbal formulas, while Ayurveda focuses on balancing bodily energies with herbs like ashwagandha (Withania somnifera) and turmeric (Curcuma longa).
- **African Traditions:** African herbal medicine is characterized by its diversity, with practices varying among different tribes and regions. It's deeply linked to spiritual beliefs and often involves using local plants like the African potato (Hypoxis hemerocallis) for various ailments.
- **European Traditions:** European herbalism has its roots in Greek and Roman medicine, evolving through the Middle Ages and Renaissance. Today, it blends traditional knowledge with modern scientific research, using herbs like lavender (Lavandula angustifolia) and chamomile (Matricaria

chamomilla).

- **Native American and Indigenous Traditions:** Native American herbal medicine uses plants like echinacea (Echinacea spp.) and goldenseal (Hydrastis canadensis). It's deeply tied to spiritual and cultural beliefs about nature and healing.

## Ancient Wisdom in Modern Times

Despite the rise of modern medicine, these ancient practices are surviving and thriving, often complementing conventional medical treatments.

- **Revival and Preservation:** There's a growing global interest in traditional herbal practices, leading to a revival and preservation of this ancient knowledge. This includes documenting traditional uses of plants and studying their effects using modern scientific methods.
- **Integration with Modern Healthcare:** In many parts of the world, traditional herbal

Medicine is being integrated into the healthcare system. For example, in China, TCM is used alongside Western medicine, and in Germany, certain herbal remedies are prescribed and regulated like conventional medicines.

## Learning from Global Herbalism

The global diversity in herbal practices provides valuable lessons for modern healthcare, offering insights into sustainable health practices and natural healing.

- **Sustainable Healthcare Practices:** Many traditional herbal practices emphasize sustainability and a holistic approach to health. For instance, the Ayurvedic principle of living in harmony with nature underscores the importance of environmental sustainability for health.
- **Cross-Cultural Exchange and Collaboration:** The increasing global

exchange of herbal knowledge fosters collaboration between traditional healers and modern researchers. This exchange enriches the global pharmacopeia and opens new health and wellness avenues.

- **Adaptation and Innovation:** Traditional practices are not static; they adapt and evolve. For example, Brazilian folk medicine now includes plants brought by enslaved Africans, demonstrating how cultural exchange can enrich herbal traditions.

## Challenges and Future Directions

The integration and preservation of global herbal traditions face several challenges and present opportunities for future development.

- **Preservation of Indigenous Knowledge:** As traditional cultures face modern pressures, there's a risk of losing indigenous knowledge. Efforts are needed to document and preserve this wisdom, respecting the intellectual property rights of indigenous communities.
- **Quality Control and Standardization:** With the globalization of herbal products, ensuring quality and standardization across different countries is challenging but essential for consumer safety and efficacy.
- **Evidence-Based Approaches:** Applying scientific methods to validate traditional uses of herbs can bridge the gap between ancient wisdom and modern science, enhancing the credibility and acceptance of herbal treatments.

Global herbal traditions represent a vast, untapped wealth of knowledge in natural healing. They offer a perspective that complements modern medicine, emphasizing a holistic, sustainable approach to health that is increasingly relevant today. As we move forward, integrating these traditions with scientific research and healthcare practices will be crucial in addressing the health challenges of the 21st century.

# CONCLUSION

As we close the pages of this first volume, "The World of Herbal Medicine," we have journeyed through the verdant fields of history, science, and global traditions.  We have seen the ancient roots of herbal healing in various cultures, traced its evolution through time, and witnessed its intersection and integration with modern medicine. This exploration has not only illuminated the depth and breadth of herbal wisdom but also underscored the vital role it continues to play in our lives today.

Understanding herbal medicine today goes beyond merely recognizing the plants and their uses.  It's about appreciating the intricacies of their active compounds, the scientific research that validates their efficacy, and the challenges and progress encountered in herbal research. This volume has aimed to provide a comprehensive understanding, comparing and contrasting the world of herbs with pharmaceuticals and showcasing their unique roles in modern medicine, including complementary and alternative health approaches.

The global herbal traditions we have explored underscore the rich cultural diversity in herbal practices, reminding us of the invaluable lessons and insights these practices offer. From the Native American to African, European, and Asian practices, each culture contributes its unique perspective, enriching the tapestry of herbal knowledge.

As we conclude this volume, remember that this journey through the world of herbal medicine is just the beginning. The subsequent volumes of "Green Healing: The Natural Medicine Bible" will delve deeper into specific aspects of herbal medicine, including cultivation techniques and the preparation of various herbal remedies like infusions, tinctures, essential oils, natural antibiotics, and much more. Each volume is a stepping stone towards mastering the art and science of herbal healing.

We invite you to continue this journey with us, further exploring the "15-in-1 Ultimate Guide: The #1 Collection of Healing Herbs and Bio-Plants to Grow, Use, and Master." The world of natural healing is vast and endlessly fascinating, and each volume of this series is designed to guide, enlighten, and inspire you on your path to wellness and a deeper understanding of the natural world.

Thank you for joining us on this journey of discovery. May the knowledge you've gained in these pages inspire you to explore further, experiment with your herbal practices, and embrace the holistic approach to health and well-being that herbal medicine offers.

# SOURCES

https://www.ncbi.nlm.nih.gov/pmc/articles/PMC3358962/

https://www.ncbi.nlm.nih.gov/pmc/articles/PMC2206236/#:~:text=Herbal%
20medicine%20is%20the%20use,standardized%20and%20tritated%20herb
al%20extracts.

https://www.medicalnewstoday.com/articles/herbal-medicine

https://www.mountsinai.org/health-library/treatment/herbal-medicine

https://www.sciencedirect.com/topics/agricultural-and-biological-sciences/
herbal-medicines

https://vitalplan.com/blogs/blog/the-science-of-herbal-medicine

https://www.ncbi.nlm.nih.gov/books/NBK92773/#:~:text=Plants%2C%20he
rbs%2C%20and%20ethnobotanicals%20have,commercial%20drug%20prep
arations%20manufactured%20today.

https://www.ncbi.nlm.nih.gov/pmc/articles/PMC6273146/

https://journals.sagepub.com/doi/pdf/10.1177/153473540200100313

https://www.who.int/news-room/feature-stories/detail/traditional-medicin

e-has-a-long-history-of-contributing-to-conventional-medicine-and-continues-to-hold-promise

https://www.sciencedirect.com/science/article/pii/S002231662214811X

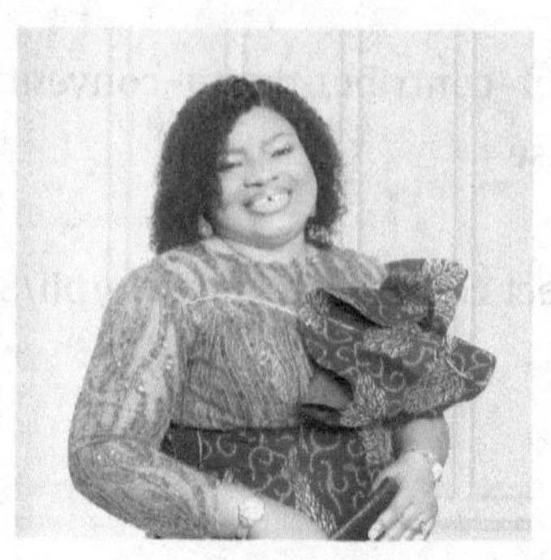

# About the Author

Glorioustina Essia is a multifaceted professional whose expertise traverses the realms of technology, artificial intelligence, literature, and natural health. As a driving force in artificial intelligence, particularly in prompt engineering, she has established herself as a pioneer. Her proficiency extends to project management, network marketing, website development, and copywriting, showcasing a unique blend of technical understanding and creative flair.

A prolific author and publisher, Glorioustina's literary works span multiple genres, captivating a diverse audience with her narrative skill and inspiring a new generation of writers to unlock their creative potential. Her passion for storytelling matches her commitment to exploring and advocating for holistic health practices. Renowned in herbal medicine, she dedicates her life to studying and promoting natural health.

Glorioustina Essia's professional and personal journey is characterized by an unwavering dedication to her core strengths and a ceaseless pursuit of knowledge. Her zeal and expertise embody the limitless possibilities that arise from a commitment to innovation, quality, and a deep-seated passion for understanding the future of technology and the ancient wisdom of herbal medicine. Glorioustina is a testament to the power of interdisciplinary knowledge and its impact in a world where technology, literature, and natural health converge.

# Also by Glorioustina Essia

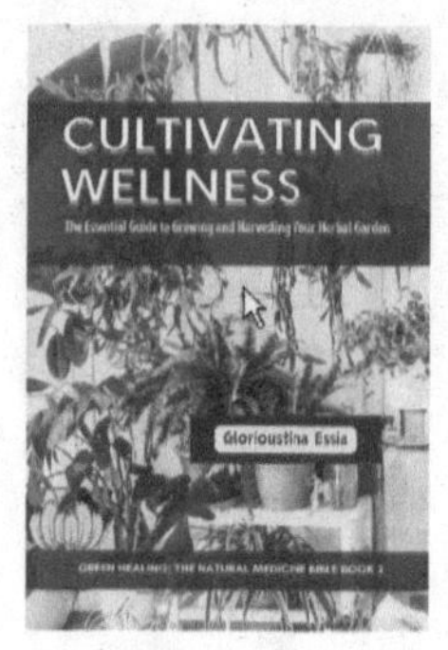

**Cultivating Wellness**

This guide is your gateway to mastering the art of herb gardening, offering practical advice for cultivating various medicinal and culinary herbs. From sustainable techniques to harvesting and preservation methods, each chapter brims with expert knowledge tailored to beginners and experienced gardeners.  Learn to navigate common challenges in herb gardening and create specialized gardens for your health and culinary needs.  Beyond gardening tips, this book inspires a deeper connection with nature and a commitment to a holistic lifestyle.  Embrace the journey of nurturing not just a garden but a healthier, more harmonious way of life with "Cultivating Wellness."

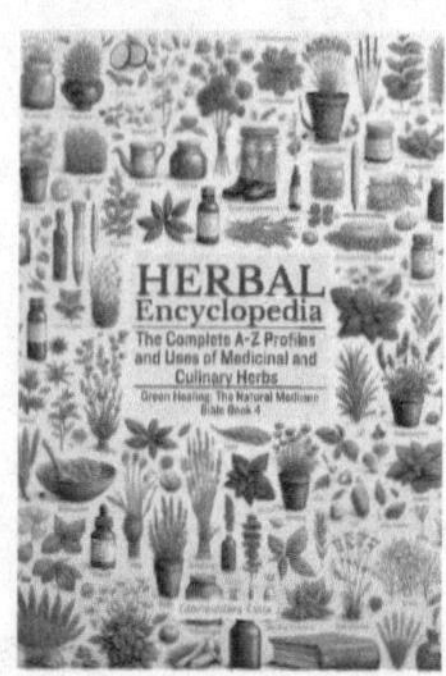

**Herbal Encyclopedia**

Embark on a journey through nature's apothecary with "Herbal Encyclopedia: The Complete A–Z Profiles and Uses of Medicinal and Culinary Herbs."  This guide unravels the secrets of herbs, from age-old medicinal uses to enhancing culinary delights.  Each page introduces you to a new herb, revealing its history, health benefits, and how it can be incorporated into your daily life. Whether you're a budding herbalist or a seasoned enthusiast, this encyclopedia offers easy-to-understand profiles, practical tips, and a connection to the ancient art of herbal healing.

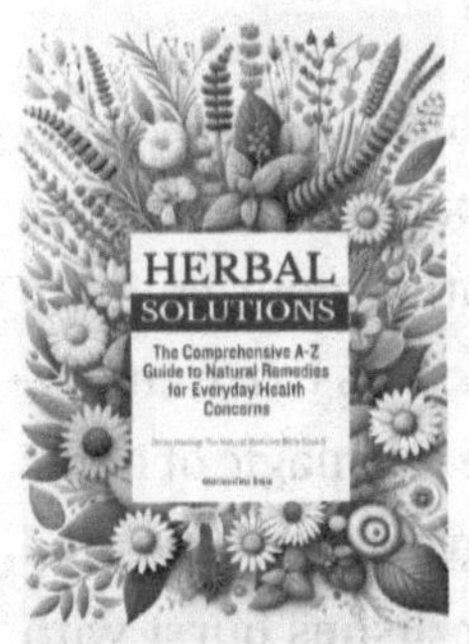

### Herbal Solutions

Discover the secrets to natural wellness with "Herbal Solutions: The Comprehensive A–Z Guide to Natural Remedies for Everyday Health Concerns" This essential resource offers easy-to-access, alphabetical listings of natural remedies for a wide range of common health issues. From herbal solutions to holistic approaches, each entry provides practical, safe, and effective ways to enhance your health naturally. Perfect for those seeking alternative options or complementing traditional medicine, this guide empowers you with the knowledge to take control of your well-being.

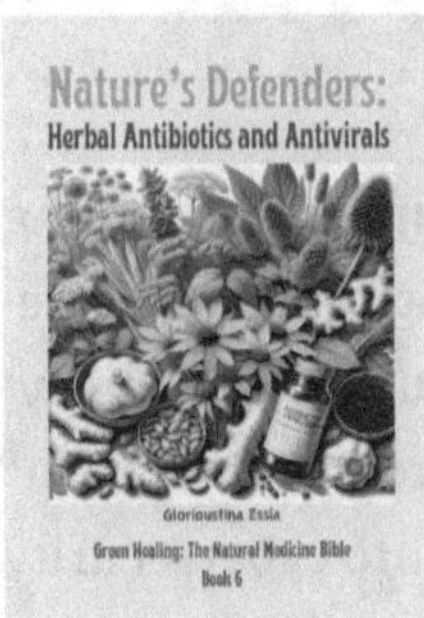

### Nature's Defenders

This essential guide unveils the power of herbal remedies in fighting infections and boosting immunity. Learn more about harnessing these natural warriors, echinacea, garlic, and elderberry, as you learn to fight against illness with natural herbs. Packed with practical advice and easy-to-follow information, this book is a must-have for anyone seeking safe, effective alternatives to conventional medicine. Embrace the wisdom of nature and discover the keys to a healthier life with "Nature's Defenders."

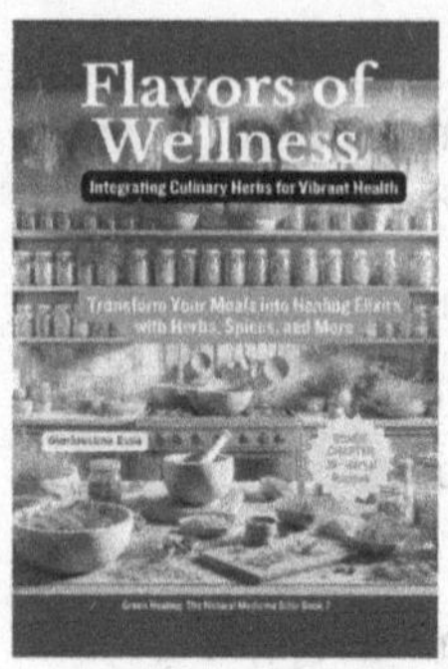

**Flavors of Wellness**

This guide invites you into a world where every herb in your garden or kitchen pantry is a key to unlocking vibrant health and elevating your culinary creations. From basil-infused breakfasts to rosemary-laced dinners, discover how to weave the magic of herbs into everyday cooking.  Learn to grow, harvest, and preserve your herbs, ensuring your dishes burst with flavor and nutritional benefits all year round. Whether you're a novice cook or a seasoned chef, this book offers simple, delicious ways to incorporate healing herbs into your daily diet. Embrace the herbal lifestyle—where wellness and flavor live harmoniously on your plate.

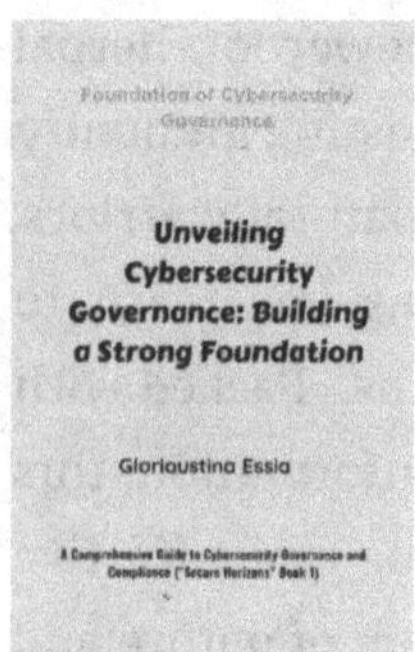

**Unveiling Cybersecurity Governance**

In the ever-expanding digital landscape, safeguarding sensitive information and maintaining robust cybersecurity practices have become paramount. "Unveiling Cybersecurity Governance: Building a Strong Foundation" is a comprehensive guide that delves into cybersecurity governance's core principles and components, equipping readers with the knowledge and tools to establish a secure digital environment.

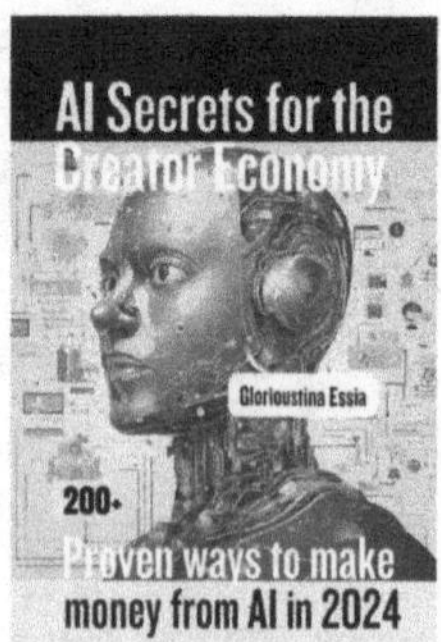

**AI Secrets for the Creator Economy: 200+ Proven ways to make money from AI in 2024**

In a world driven by innovation and transformation, the Creator Economy emerges as a powerful force, with Artificial Intelligence (AI) at its beating heart.  This book, "AI Secrets for the Creator Economy: 200+ Proven Ways to Make Money from AI in 2024 and Beyond," is more than just a book; it's your key to unlocking the incredible synergy between AI and creativity, opening the door to a wealth of opportunities for those who are willing to seize them.